Women's Health Mnemonics for the Nurse Practitioner

By Nachole Johnson

Illustrations by Murhiel Cabarte

ISBN-13: 978-1974124879
ISBN-10: 1974124878
Printed in the United States of America
10 9 8 7 6 5 4 3 2 1

Why I Wrote This Book

There's a lot to learn while you are in nurse practitioner school. Because of the time pressure, I really appreciated anything that would help me get through school. I've always been a visual learner, and it is easy for me to pick up information if I draw out pictures or play with words to make learning a complex issue easier. I loved using mnemonics when I was in nursing school, and that continued when I went to graduate school for my Family Nurse Practitioner degree.

I found it was easy for me to remember silly sayings during the test that would remind me of the right answer. Turns out, many other people like mnemonics too! I decided to write a book specifically for the nurse practitioner field. Women's Health Mnemonics for the Nurse Practitioner is a general guide to women's health, meaning it will help you in school and out.

Use this book as a guide to memorize common concepts and as a refresher for ones you haven't used in a while. Even when you are out of school and in practice, it is sometimes difficult to remember a concept you haven't used since the final exam. This is normal, and happens to nurse practitioners and physicians alike. I still use silly mnemonics to remember things like the cranial nerves, "**O**n **O**ld **O**lympus **T**owering **T**ops **A** **F**in **A**nd **G**erman **V**iewed **S**ome **H**ops," anyone?

Use this book while you are in school and as a refresher when you finish. I've included extras for Nurse Practitioners like common obstetrical and gynecology abbreviations, terminology, and early childhood milestones. Have fun, learn, and enjoy!

Nachole

TABLE OF CONTENTS

Chapter 1
Obstetric and Gynecology Abbreviations

AB - abortion; may see SAB (spontaneous) or TAB (therapeutic) or EAB (elective)

AC - abdominal circumference (sono)

AFI - amnionic fluid index (sono); normal = 5 to 20

AGA - appropriate for gestational age

BPD - biparietal diameter (sono)

Chl - chlamydia, usually referring to gen probe

Ctx - contractions

CVAT - costovetebral angle tenderness, a symptom of pyelonephritis

DM - diabetes mellitus, may also see GDM (gestational)

DR - delivery room

EBL - estimated blood loss

EDC - estimated date of confinement (due date)

EFW - estimated fetal weight (sono)

FBS - fasting blood sugar

FFN - fetal fibronectin

FH - fundal height

FHT - fetal heart tones

FOC - father of child

FTG - Foley to gravity

GA - gestational age

GIFT - gamete intrafallopian transfer

G#P# - gravida, para

G - total # of pregnancies

P - total # of delivered pregnancies

T - total # of term deliveries (after 37 weeks)

P - total # of preterm deliveries (20-36 weeks)

A - total # of abortions/miscarriages (before 20 weeks)

L - total # of living children

* Note: for TPA twins count as one number, but for L they count as two

HSG- hysterosalpingography

HTN - hypertension, may see CHTN (chronic)

HBsAg - Hepatitis B surface Antigen

HGSIL - high grade squamous intraepithelial lesion

IAL - in active labor; may see NIAL (not)

ICSI - intracytoplasmic sperm injection

IDC - indirect Coomb's test

IUI- intrauterine insemination

IUP - intrauterine pregnancy; may see PTIUP (preterm), TIUP (term)

IVDA - intravenous drug abuse

IUFD - intrauterine fetal demise

IVF-ET - in vitro fertilization with embryo transfer

L/C/P - long, closed, posterior cervical exam when a woman is not in labor

LGA - large for gestational age

LGSIL - low grade squamous intraepithelial lesion

LMP - last menstrual period (first day of)

LTCS - low transverse cesarean section; refers to type of incision on the uterus and not the skin

MGA - mean gestational age (sono)

MI - menstrual index: age of patient at 1st period/cycle length/duration of period

MLE - midline episiotomy, usually preceded by degree, e.g. 2° MLE

MMR - measles, mumps, rubella vaccine; given to rubella sensitive patients post-partum

MSAFP - maternal serum alpha feto protein; prenatal test for Down's, if increased positive for neural tube defects if decreased - screening test only

NST - non-stress test; classified as NST-NR (non-reactive) or NST-R (reactive)

NTD - neural tube defect; e.g. meningomyelocele, spina bifida

NMDC - no malignant or dysplastic cells; pap smear results

OCP - oral contraceptive pill; also written BCP (birth control pill)

PID - pelvic inflammatory disease

PML - preterm (premature) labor

PNV - prenatal vitamins

POD# - post op day #

PPD# - post partum day #

ROM - rupture of membranes (broken bag of water); may see AROM (artificial), PROM (preterm = less than 37 weeks), SROM (spontaneous), PPROM (preterm, premature = 12 to 24 hours before labor starts)

Rub - rubella, usually refers to the titer

SGA - small for gestational age

STD - sexually transmitted disease

SVD - spontaneous vaginal delivery (no forceps or vacuum)

TOL - trial of labor

3VC - three-vessel cord

VBAC - vaginal birth after c-section

WBD - weeks by dates (by LMP)

Chapter 2
Obstetric Medical Terminology

G= Gravida means # of Pregnancy
P= Parity means # of deliveries > 20 weeks , Ptpal
(T=term,preterm,abortion, live child)
Term= > 37 wks,< 42 wks, or >2500 gms
Preterm= 20-37 wks,>500 gms <2500gms
Abortion= <20 weeks, <500gms,<25cm
Post term= >42 weeks
Puerperium= birth - 42 days postpartum
Trimesters: 1st <12 wks, 2nd = 13-28 wks, 3rd = >28 wks

Amenorrhea - absence or cessation of menstrual periods.

Amenorrhea, primary - from the beginning and lifelong; menstruation never begins at puberty.

Amenorrhea, secondary - due to some physical cause and usually of later onset; a condition in which menstrual periods which were at one time normal and regular become increasing abnormal and irregular or absent.

Anovulation - failure of the ovaries to produce or release mature eggs.

Benign - cell growth that is not cancerous, does not invade nearby tissue, or spread to other parts of the body.

Biological therapy (also called immunotherapy, biotherapy, or biological response modifier therapy) - uses the body's immune system, either directly or indirectly, to fight cancer or to lessen side effects that may be caused by some cancer treatments.

Biopsy - removal of sample of tissue via a hollow needle or scalpel.

Cancer - abnormal cells that divide without control, which can invade nearby tissues or spread through the bloodstream and lymphatic system to other parts of the body.

Carcinogen - a substance that is known to cause cancer.

Certified nurse midwife - an individual educated in the two disciplines of nursing and midwifery who provides care of normal newborns and women before and during pregnancy, in labor, and after delivery.

Cervicitis - an irritation of the cervix by a number of different organisms. Cervicitis is generally classified as either acute or chronic.

Cervix - the lower, narrow part of the uterus (womb) located between the bladder and the rectum. It forms a canal that opens into the vagina, which leads to the outside of the body.

Chemotherapy - treatment to destroy cancer cells with drugs.

Chlamydial infection - very common sexually transmitted disease or urinary tract infection caused by a bacteria-like organism in the urethra and reproductive system.

Climacteric (also called perimenopause) - the transition period of time before menopause, marked by a decreased production of estrogen and progesterone, irregular menstrual periods, and transitory psychological changes.

Clinical trials - organized research studies that provide clinical data aimed at finding better ways to prevent, detect, diagnose, or treat diseases.

Cold knife cone biopsy - a procedure in which a laser or a surgical scalpel is used to remove a piece of tissue. This procedure requires the use of general anesthesia.

Colony-stimulating factors - substances that stimulate the production of blood cells.

Colposcopy (also called colposcopic biopsy) - a procedure which uses an instrument with magnifying lenses, called a colposcope, to examine the cervix for abnormalities. If abnormal tissue is found, a biopsy is usually performed.

Computed tomography (also called CT or CAT scan) - a noninvasive procedure that takes cross-sectional images of the brain or other internal organs; to detect any abnormalities that may not show up on an ordinary X-ray. The CT scan may indicate enlarged lymph nodes - a possible sign of a spreading cancer or of an infection.

Cone biopsy (also called conization) - a biopsy in which a larger cone-shaped piece of tissue is removed from the cervix by using the loop electrosurgical excision procedure or the cold knife cone biopsy procedure. The cone biopsy procedure may be used as a treatment for precancerous lesions and early cancers.

Cryosurgery - use of liquid nitrogen, or a probe that is very cold, to freeze and kill cancer cells.

Culdocentesis - a procedure in which a needle is inserted into the pelvic cavity through the vaginal wall to obtain a sample of fluid.

Cyst - a fluid-filled or semi-solid sac in or under the skin.

Cystitis - inflammation of the urinary bladder and ureters.

Dilation and curettage (also called D & C) - a minor operation in which the cervix is dilated (expanded) so that the cervical canal and uterine lining can be scraped with a curette (spoon-shaped instrument).

Dysmenorrhea - pain or discomfort experienced just before or during a menstrual period.

Dysmenorrhea, primary - from the beginning and usually lifelong; severe and frequent menstrual cramping caused by uterine contractions.

Dysmenorrhea, secondary - due to some physical cause and usually of later onset; painful menstrual periods caused by another medical condition present in the body (i.e., pelvic inflammatory disease, endometriosis).

Dyspareunia - pain in the vagina or pelvis experienced during sexual intercourse.

Ectopic pregnancy (also called tubal pregnancy) - pregnancy that develops outside the uterus, usually in one of the fallopian tubes.

Endocervical curettage (ECC) - a procedure which uses a narrow instrument called a curette to scrape the lining of the endocervical canal. This type of biopsy is usually completed along with the colposcopic biopsy.

Endometrial ablation - a procedure to destroy the lining of the uterus (endometrium).

Endometrial biopsy - a procedure in which a sample of tissue is obtained through a tube which is inserted into the uterus.

Endometrial hyperplasia - abnormal thickening of the endometrium caused by excessive cell growth.

Endometrial implants - fragments of endometrium that relocate outside of the uterus, such as in the muscular wall of the uterus, ovaries, fallopian tubes, vagina, or intestine.

Endometrial resection - a procedure to remove the lining of the uterus (endometrium).

Endometriosis - condition in which tissue resembling that of the endometrium grows outside the uterus, on or near the ovaries or fallopian tubes, or in other areas of the pelvic cavity.

Endometrium - mucous membrane lining of the inner surface of the uterus that grows during each menstrual cycle and is shed in menstrual blood.

Endoscopy - use of a very flexible tube with a lens or camera (and a light on the end), which is connected to a computer screen, allowing the provider to see inside the hollow organs, such as the uterus. Biopsy samples can be taken through the tube.

Estrogen - a group of hormones secreted by the ovaries which affect many aspects of the female body, including a woman's menstrual cycle and normal sexual and reproductive development.

Estrogen replacement therapy (ERT) - use of the female hormone estrogen to replace that which the body no longer produces naturally after medical or surgical menopause.

Excisional - cutting away cancerous tissue with a scalpel or other instruments to completely remove it and possibly some surrounding tissue. There are many types of excisional surgeries, each named for the particular area of the body in which they are performed or the particular purpose for which they are performed.

Expectant management (also called expectant therapy) - "watchful waiting" or close monitoring of a disease by a doctor instead of immediate treatment.

Extragenital - outside of, away from, unrelated to the genital organs.

Fallopian tubes - two thin tubes that extend from each side of the uterus, toward the ovaries, as a passageway for eggs and sperm.

Family nurse practitioner - a nurse with advanced education to provide direct health care to children, women, and men.

Fecal occult blood test - test to check for hidden blood in stool.

Fertile - able to become pregnant.

Fibroids - noncancerous growths in, on, or within the walls of the uterus.

Fibroid embolization - a minimally-invasive (without a large abdominal incision) technique which involves identifying which arteries are supplying blood to the fibroids and then blocking off these arteries, which cuts off the fibroids blood supply and causes them to shrink. Researchers are still evaluating the long-term implications of this procedure on fertility and regrowth of the fibroid.

Follicle-stimulating hormone (FSH) - hormone secreted by the pituitary gland in the brain that stimulates the growth and maturation of eggs in females and sperm in males, and sex hormone production in both males and females.

Genital herpes - a sexually transmitted disease caused by the herpes simplex virus.

Genital warts - a sexually transmitted disease caused by the human papillomavirus (HPV).

Genitals - external sex organs.

Grading - a process for classifying cancer cells to determine the growth rate of the tumor. The cancer cells are measured by how closely they look like normal cells.

Hirsutism - excess growth of body and facial hair, including the chest, stomach, and back.

Hormone therapy (HT) - use of the female hormones estrogen and progestin (a synthetic form of progesterone) to treat symptoms that result when those hormones are no longer produced in menopause; also used as treatment of cancer by removing, blocking, or adding hormones.

Hormones - chemical substances created by the body that control numerous body functions.

Human papillomaviruses (HPVs) - a group of viruses that can cause warts. Some HPVs are sexually transmitted and cause wart-like growths on the genitals. HPV is associated with some types of cancer.

Hyperplasia - an abnormal increase in the number of cells in a tissue or an organ (i.e., cervix or the lining of the uterus).

Hysterectomy - surgery to remove the uterus.

Hysterosalpingography - X-ray examination of the uterus and fallopian tubes that uses dye and is often performed to rule out tubal obstruction.

Hysteroscopy - visual examination of the canal of the cervix and the interior of the uterus using a viewing instrument (hysteroscope) inserted through the vagina.

Imaging - tests or evaluation procedures that produce pictures of areas inside the body.

Immune system - group of organs, antibodies, and cells that defends the body against infection or disease.

Immunotherapy (also called biological therapy) - treatment that uses the body's natural defenses to fight cancer.

Infertility - not being able to produce children.

Interferon - a biological response modifier that stimulates the growth of certain disease-fighting blood cells in the immune system.

Interleukin-2 - a biological response modifier that stimulates the growth of certain blood cells in the immune system that can fight cancer.

Invasive cancer - cancer that begins in one area and then spreads deeper into the tissues of that area.

Labia - the folds of skin at the opening of the vagina (and other organs).

Laparoscopic lymph node sampling - lymph nodes are removed through a viewing tube called a laparoscope, which is inserted through a small incision in the abdomen.

Laparoscopy - use of a viewing tube with a lens or camera (and a light on the end), which is inserted through a small incision in the abdomen to examine the contents of the abdomen and remove tissue samples.

Laparotomy - a surgical procedure that involves an incision from the upper to lower abdomen; often used when making a diagnosis by less invasive tests is difficult.

Loop electrosurgical excision procedure (LEEP) - a procedure which uses an electric wire loop to obtain a piece of tissue.

Luteinizing hormone (LH) - hormone secreted by the pituitary gland in the brain that stimulates the growth and maturation of eggs in females and sperm in males.

Lymph nodes (also called lymph glands) - small organs located in the channels of the lymphatic system which store special cells to trap bacteria or cancer cells traveling through the body in lymph. Clusters of lymph nodes are found in the underarms, groin, neck, chest, and abdomen.

Lymphatic system - tissues and organs, including bone marrow, spleen, thymus, and lymph nodes, that produce, store, and carry white blood cells to fight infection and disease.

Magnetic resonance imaging (MRI) - a noninvasive procedure that produces a two-dimensional view of an internal organ or structure, especially the brain and spinal cord. The MRI may show abnormal nodules in bones or lymph nodes - a sign that cancer may be spreading.

Malignant - cancerous cells are present.

Mammogram - X-ray of the breast tissue.

Menarche - a young woman's first menstrual period.

Menopause - end of menstruation; commonly used to refer to the period ending the female reproductive phase of life.

Menorrhagia - the most common type of abnormal uterine bleeding (also called dysfunctional uterine bleeding) characterized by heavy and prolonged menstrual bleeding. In some cases, bleeding may be so severe and relentless that daily activities become interrupted.

Menses - menstrual flow.

Menstruation - a cyclical process of the endometrium shedding its lining, along with discharge from the cervix and vagina, from the vaginal opening. This process results from the mature egg cell (ovum) not being fertilized by a sperm cell as it travels from one of the ovaries down a fallopian tube to the uterus, in the process called ovulation.

Metastasis - spread of cancer from one part of the body to another.

Metrorrhagia - any irregular, acyclical nonmenstrual bleeding from the uterus; bleeding between menstrual periods.

Monoclonal antibodies - substances that can locate and bind to cancer cells wherever they are in the body.

Obstetrician/gynecologist (OB/GYN) - a doctor who specializes in general women's medical care, diagnosis and treatment of disorders of the female reproductive system, and care of pregnant women.

Oligomenorrhea - infrequent or light menstrual cycles.

Oncologist - a doctor who specializes in treating cancer.

Oophorectomy - surgery to remove one or both ovaries.

Ovaries - two female reproductive organs located in the pelvis.

Ovulation - release of a mature egg from an ovary.

Ovum - a mature egg cell released during ovulation from an ovary.

Pap test (also called Pap smear) - test that involves microscopic examination of cells collected from the cervix, used to detect changes that may be cancer or may lead to cancer, and to show noncancerous conditions, such as infection or inflammation.

Pathologist - a doctor who identifies diseases by studying cells and tissues under a microscope.

Pelvic examination - an internal examination of the uterus, vagina, ovaries, fallopian tubes, bladder, and rectum.

Pelvic inflammatory disease (PID) - inflammation of the pelvic organs caused by a type of bacteria.

Pelvic lymph node dissection - removal of some lymph nodes from the pelvis.

Pelvis - a basin-shaped structure that supports the spinal column and contains the sacrum, coccyx, and hip bones (ilium, pubis, and ischium).

Perimenopause (also called climacteric) - the transition period of time before menopause, marked by a decreased production of estrogen and progesterone, irregular menstrual periods, and transitory psychological changes.

Perineal - related to the perineum.

Perineum - area between the anus and the sex organs.

Peripheral stem cell support - procedure to replace blood-forming cells destroyed by cancer treatment. Stem cells in the blood that are similar to cells in the bone marrow are removed from the patient's blood before treatment and given back to the patient after treatment.

Placenta - organ that develops in the uterus during pregnancy; links the blood supplies of a pregnant woman to the fetus to provide nutrients and remove waste products.

Polymenorrhea - too frequent menstruation.

Polyps - a growth that projects from the lining of mucous membrane, such as the intestine.

Postmenopausal bleeding - any bleeding that occurs more than six months after the last normal menstrual period at menopause.

Premenstrual dysphoric disorder (PMDD) - a much more severe form of the collective symptoms known as premenstrual syndrome (PMS), premenstrual dysphoric disorder (PMDD) is considered a severe and chronic medical condition that requires attention and treatment.

Premenstrual syndrome (PMS) - a group of physical and emotional symptoms that some women experience during their menstrual cycle. Although the symptoms usually cease with onset of the menstrual period, in some women, symptoms may last through and after their menstrual periods.

Progesterone - female hormone.

Progestin - synthetic form of the female sex hormone progesterone.

Radiation therapy (also called radiotherapy) - treatment with high-energy rays (such as X-rays or gamma rays) to kill cancer cells; may be by external radiation or by internal radiation from radioactive materials placed directly in or near the tumor.

Radionuclide scan - an imaging scan in which a small amount of radioactive substance is injected into the vein. A machine measures levels of radioactivity in certain organs, thereby detecting any abnormal areas or tumors.

Rectum - lower end of the large intestine, leading to the anus.

Recur - to occur again; reappearance of cancer cells at the same site or in another location.

Risk factor - activity or factor that may increase the chance of developing a disease.

Salpingectomy - surgical removal of one or both fallopian tubes.

Salpingo-oophorectomy - surgery to remove the fallopian tubes and ovaries.

Schiller test - a diagnostic test in which the cervix is coated with an iodine solution to detect the presence of abnormal cells.

Sexually transmitted disease (STD) - infection spread through sexual intercourse and other intimate sexual contact.

Screening - checking for disease when there are no symptoms.

Stage - the extent of a cancer, whether the disease has spread from the original site to other parts of the body.

Surgery - operation to remove or repair a part of the body, or to find out if disease is present.

Systemic treatment - treatment using substances that travel through the bloodstream and reach cancer cells all over the body.

Tamoxifen - an anticancer drug used in hormone therapy to block the effects of estrogen.

Tissue - group or layer of cells that together perform specific functions.

Total hysterectomy - the removal of the uterus, including the cervix; the fallopian tubes and the ovaries remain.

Total hysterectomy with bilateral salpingo-oophorectomy - the entire uterus, fallopian tubes, and the ovaries are surgically removed.

Transvaginal ultrasound (also called ultrasonography) - an ultrasound test using a small instrument, called a transducer, that is placed in the vagina.

Trichomoniasis - very common type of vaginitis caused by a single-celled organism usually transmitted during sexual contact.

Tumor - abnormal mass of tissue that results from excessive cell division; may be benign (not cancerous) or malignant (cancerous).

Ultrasound - an imaging technique that uses sound waves to produce an image on a monitor of the abdominal organs, such as the uterus, liver, and kidneys.

Urethra - narrow channel through which urine passes from the bladder out of the body.

Urethritis - infection limited to the urethra.

Uterus - also called the womb, the uterus is a hollow, pear-shaped organ located in a woman's lower abdomen, between the bladder and the rectum.

Vagina (also called the birth canal) - the passageway through which fluid passes out of the body during menstrual periods. The vagina connects the cervix (the opening of the womb, or uterus) and the vulva (the external genitalia).

Vaginal atrophy - often a symptom of menopause; the drying and thinning of the tissues of the vagina and urethra. This can lead to dyspareunia (pain during sexual intercourse) as well as vaginitis, cystitis, and urinary tract infections.

Vaginal hysterectomy - the uterus is removed through the vaginal opening.

Vaginitis - inflammation, redness, or swelling of the vaginal tissues; usually resulting from a bacterial infection.

Vaginitis, atrophic - a form of noninfectious vaginitis which usually results from a decrease in hormones because of menopause, surgical removal of the ovaries, radiation therapy, or even after childbirth - particularly in breastfeeding women. Lack of estrogen dries and thins the vaginal tissue, and may also cause spotting.

Vaginitis, bacterial - very common vaginal infection characterized by symptoms such as increased vaginal discharge or itching, burning, or redness in the genital area.

Vaginitis, noninfectious - a type of vaginitis that usually refers to vaginal irritation without an infection being present. Most often, the infection is caused by an allergic reaction to, or irritation from, vaginal sprays, douches, or spermicidal products. It may also be caused by sensitivity to perfumed soaps, detergents, or fabric softeners.

Vaginitis, viral - very common vaginal infection, often sexually transmitted, that is caused by one of many different types of viruses (i.e., herpes simplex virus, human papillomavirus).

Vulva - external, visible part of the female genital area.

Vulvitis - an inflammation of the vulva, the soft folds of skin outside the vagina. This is not a condition but rather a symptom that results from a host of diseases, infections, injuries, allergies, and other irritants.

White blood cells - cells that help the body fight infection and disease.

X-ray - electromagnetic energy used to produce images of bones and internal organs onto film.

Yeast infection (also called Candida) - one type of vaginitis caused by the Candida fungus characterized by itching, burning, or redness of the vaginal area.

Chapter 3
The Menstrual Cycle

Menstrual Cycle
"FOL(d) M(a)PS"

Ovarian cycle:
Follicular phase, **O**vulatory phase, **L**uteal phase

Menstrual cycle:
Menstrual flow, **P**roliferative phase, **S**ecretory phase

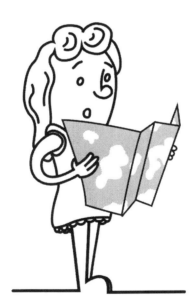

The ovarian cycle controls the menstrual cycle. The cycle begins (day 0) when menstrual flow starts. At day 14, the luteal and secretory phases begin and last until day 28, after which the cycle begins again.

Normal Numbers for gestation period, oocytes, vaginal pH and menstrual cycle

"Rule of 4"

4 is the normal pH of the vagina.

40 weeks is the normal gestation period.

400 oocytes released between menarche and menopause.

400,000 oocytes present at puberty.

28 days in a normal menstrual cycle.

280 days (from last normal menstrual period) in a normal gestation period.

Causes of secondary amenorrhea
"SOAP"

Stress

OCP

Anorexia

Pregnancy

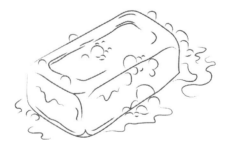

Menopause symptoms:
"FSH > 20 IU/L"

FSH is the most accurate blood test for confirmation of menopause!
· **F**lushes (hot) /**F**emale genitalia (vaginal) dryness and burning
· **S**weats at night
· **H**eadaches
· **I**nsomnia
· **U**rge incontinence
· **L**ibido decreases

Sexual response cycle
"EXPLORE"

EXcitement
PLateau
Orgasmic
REsolution

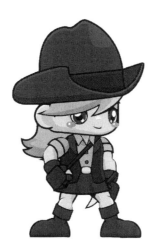

Premenopausal symptoms
"HAVOC"

Hot flashes
Atrophy of vagina
Vaginal dryness
Osteoporosis
CAD

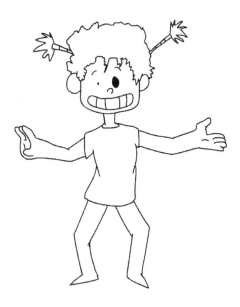

3 major causes of Dysfunctional uterine bleeding "DUB"

Don't ovulate (anovulation: 90% of cases)
Unusual corpus leuteum activity (prolonged or insufficient)
Birth control pills (since they increase progesterone-estrogen ratio)

Anterior Pituitary Hormones "FLAGTOP"

F: Follicle Stimulating Hormone
L: Luteinizing Hormone
A: ACTH
G: Growth Hormone
T: Thyroid Stimulating Hormone
O: MSH - melanOcyte stimulating hormone
P: Prolactin

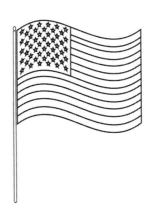

Role of FSH and LH

FSH

In women, FSH stimulates ovarian follicles (which secrete estrogen, which stimulates endometrial proliferation).

LH

In women, LH stimulates corpus luteum→ women have "**L**ittle **H**ips and **C**ute **L**egs"

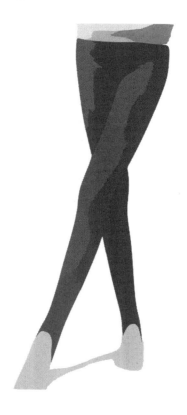

Corpus luteum secretes estrogen and progesterone, which stimulates the endometrium

Chapter 4
CONTRACEPTIVES

Oral contraceptive complications and warning signs
"ACHES"

Abdominal pain
Chest pain
Headache (severe)
Eye (blurred vision)
Sharp leg pain

Side effects of oral contraceptives
"CONTRACEPTIVES"

Cholestatic jaundice
Oedema (corneal)
Nasal congestion
Thyroid dysfunction
Raised BP
Acne/ **A**lopecia/ **A**nemia
Cerebrovascular disease
Elevated blood sugar
Porphyria/ **P**igmentation/ **P**ancreatitis
Thromboembolism
Intracranial hypertension
Vomiting (progesterone only)
Erythema nodosum/ **E**xtrapyramidal effects
Sensitivity to light

Serious complications of oral birth control pills
"SEA CASH"

Severe leg pain
Eye problems
Abdominal problems

Chest pain
Acne
Swelling of ankles and feet
Headaches (severe)

IUD side effects
"PAINS"

Period that is late
Abdominal cramps
Increase in body temperature
Noticeable vaginal discharge
Spotting

Chapter 5
ABDOMINAL PAIN/DISORDERS

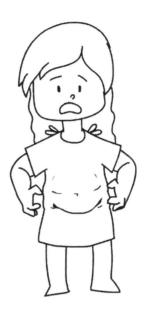

Asherman syndrome features
"ASHERMAN"

Acquired Anomaly
Secondary to Surgery
Hysterosalpingography confirms diagnosis
Endometrial damage/ **E**ugonadotropic
Repeated uterine trauma
Missed Menses
Adhesions
Normal estrogen and progesterone

Causes of abdominal pain during pregnancy
"LARA CROFT"

Labor
Abruption of placenta
Rupture (eg. ectopic/ uterus)
Abortion

Cholestasis
Rectus sheath haematoma
Ovarian tumour
Fibroids
Torsion of uterus

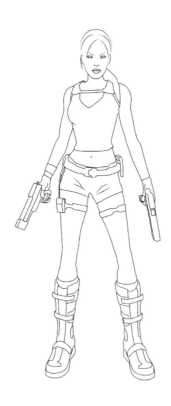

RLQ pain
"AEIOU"

Appendicitis/ **A**bscess
Ectopic pregnancy/ **E**ndometriosis
Inflammatory disease (pelvic)/ **I**BD
Ovarian cyst (rupture, torsion)
Uteric colic/ **U**rinary stones

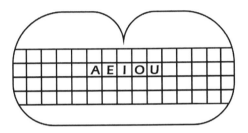

Pelvic Inflammatory Disease (PID) causes and effects
"PID CAN be EPIC"

Causes:
Chlamydia trachomatis
Actinomycetes
Neisseria gonorrhoeae

Effects:
Ectopic
Pregnancy
Infertility
Chronic pain

Pelvic Inflammatory Disease (PID) complications "I FACE PID"

Infertility

Fitz-Hugh-Curtis syndrome
Abscesses
Chronic pelvic pain
Ectopic pregnancy

Peritonitis
Intestinal obstruction
Disseminated: sepsis, endocarditis, arthritis, meninigitis

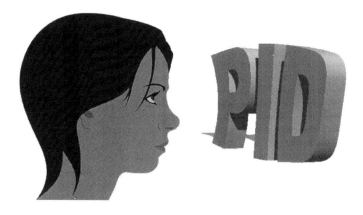

Ovarian cancer risk factors
"B FILM"

Breast cancer
Family history
Infertility
Low parity
Mumps

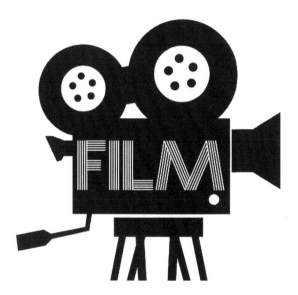

Omental caking

Omental **CA**king = **O**varian **CA**

"Omental caking" is the term for ascities, plus a fixed upper abdominal and pelvic mass. It almost always signifies ovarian cancer.

First line treatment for Polycystic Ovarian Syndrome (PCOS)

Treat PCOS with OCP's (oral contraceptive pills).

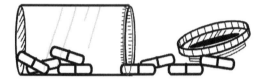

Chapter 6
PREGNANCY

Prenatal care questions
"ABCDEF"

Amniotic fluid leakage?
Bleeding vaginally?
Contractions?
Dysuria?
Edema?
Fetal movement?

PRENATAL DIAGNOSTIC
Timing

U-CAT

U..........USG..............6-40WKS.
C..........CVS..............10-14
A..........AMNIOCENTESIS..15-17
T..........TRIPLE TEST.......15-18

Diagnostic tests
"CAT"

C=CHORIONI VILOOUS SAMPLING=10-14wks of gestation
A=AMINOCENTESIS=15-17wks. of gestation
T=Triple test(MSAFP)= 15-18wks of gestation

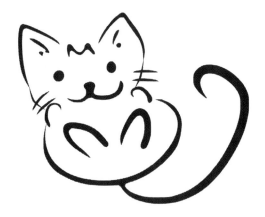

Bleeding During Pregnancy
"APH"

Abruptio placentae
Placenta previa
Hemorrhage from the GU tract

IUGR causes

IUGR
Inherited: chromosomal and genetic disorders
Uterus: placental insufficiency
General: maternal malnutrition, smoking
Rubella and other congenital infection

Classic triad of Preeclampsia

PREeclampsia
Proteinuria
Rising blood pressure
Edema

Placenta-crossing Substances
"WANT My Hot Dog"

Wastes
Antibodies
Nutrients
Teratogens
Microorganisms
Hormones, **H**IV
Drugs

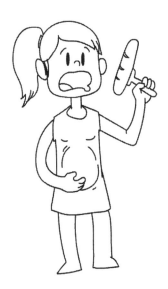

When CVS and amniocentesis are performed

When performed:
"Chorionic V" has
10 letters and Chorionic villus sampling is performed at
10 weeks gestation.

"AlphaFetoProtein" has
16 letters and is measured at
16 weeks gestation.

Causes for increased maternal serum Alpha-fetoprotein (AFP) during pregnancy

"Increased **M**aternal **S**erum **A**lpha **F**eto **P**rotein"
Intestinal obstruction
Multiple gestation/ **M**iscalculation of gestational age/ **M**yeloschisis
Spina bifida cystica
Anencephaly/ Abdominal wall defect
Fetal death
Placental abruption

Major causes for increased maternal serum Alpha-fetoprotein (AFP) during pregnancy

TOLD
Testicular tumours
Obituary (fetal death)
Liver: hepatomas
Defects (neural tube defects)

Neonatal vitamin toxicities

Excess vitamin **A**: **A**nomalies (teratogenic)
Excess vitamin **E**: **E**nterocolitis (necrotizing enterocolitis)
Excess vitamin **K**: **K**ernicterus (hemolysis)

Chapter 7
CHILD BIRTH

Indication for forceps delivery
"FORCEPS"

Fetus alive
Os dilated
Ruptured membrane
Cervix taken up
Engagement of head
Presentation suitable
Sagittal suture in AP diameter of inlet

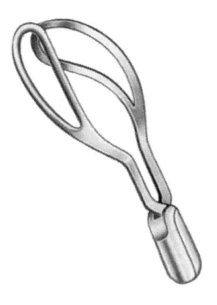

Instrumental delivery prerequisites
"AABBCCDDEE"

Analgesia
Antisepsis
Bowel empty
Bladder empty
Cephalic presentation
Consent
Dilated cervix
Disproportion (no CPD)
Engaged
Episiotomy

FORCEPS/VACUUM DELIVERY "ABCDEFGHHIJ"

A - Anesthesia/Assistance (anesthetist, colleague,pediatrician)
Think and prepare for shoulder dystocia
B- Bladder empty
C- Cervix fully dilated
D- determine position
E- Explain to the patient/ exit plan if it fails, ready for cesarean section
F - Fontanelle (to check position)
G - Gentle traction
H- Handle elevated for forceps
Halt for vacuum (no descent with 3 pulls, 3 times pop off)
I - Incision/Episiotomy
J- remove forceps when jaw visible

Indications for early cord clamping
"RAPID CS"

Rh incompatibility
Asphyxia
Premature delivery
Infections
Diabetic mother
CS (cesarean section) previously, so the funda is RAPID CS

Post-partum hemorrhage risk factors
"PARTUM"

Polyhydroamnios/ Prolonged labor/ Previous cesarean
APH/ ANTH
Recent bleeding history
Twins
Uterine fibroids
Multiparity

Episiotomy assessment
"REEDA"

Redness
Edema
Ecchymosis
Discharge, drainage
Approximation

Post-partum hemorrhage causes
"4T's"

Tissue (retained placenta)
Tone (uterine atony)
Trauma (traumatic delivery, episiotomy)
Thrombin (coagulation disorders, DIC)

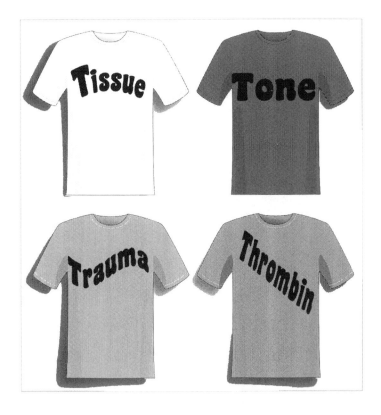

Infertility causes and risk factors
"INFERTILE"

Idiopathic
No ovulation – PCOS, menopause, pituitary disease, thyroid disorders
Fibroids – physical hindrance
Endometriosis
Regular bleeding pattern disrupted – oligo/amenorrhoea
Tubal disease leading to blocked/damaged cilia
Increasing age >35 years
Large size – obesity
Excessive weight loss – anorexia nervosa

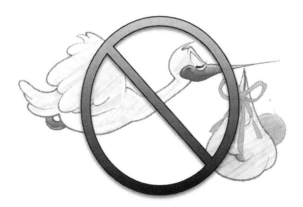

B-agonist tocolytic contraindications or warnings
"ABCDE"

Angina (Heart disease)
BP high
Chorioamnionitis
Diabetes

Excessive bleeding

Female pelvis shapes
"GAP"

In order from the most to least common:
Gynecoid
Android /**A**nthropoid
Platypelloid

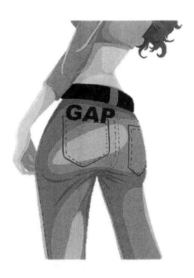

Causes of postpartum collapse
"HEPARINS"

Hemorrhage
Eclampsia
Pulmonary embolism
Amniotic fluid embolism
Regional anaesthetic complications
Infarction (MI)

Neurogenic shock
Septic shock

Complications of Multiple pregnancies
"HI, PAPA"

Hydramnios (Poly)
IUGR

Preterm labour
Antepartum haemorrhage
Pre-eclampsia
Abortion

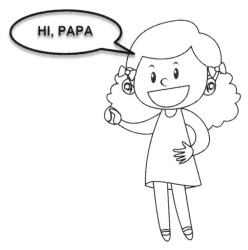

Preterm labor causes
"DISEASE"

Dehydration
Infection

Sex
Exercise (strenuous)
Activities
Stress
Environmental factor (job, etc)

Recurrent miscarriage causes
"RIBCAGE"

Radiation
Immune reaction
Bugs (infection)
Cervical incompetence
Anatomical anomaly (uterine septum etc.)
Genetic (aneuploidy, balanced translocation etc.)
Endocrine

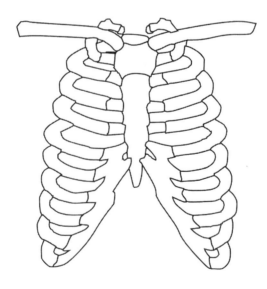

Management of shoulder dystocia:
"HELPERRR"

call for **H**elp
Episiotomy
Legs up [McRoberts position]
Pressure suprapubically [not on fundus]
Enter vagina for shoulder rotation
Reach for posterior shoulder and deliver posterior shoulder/
Return head into vagina [Zavanelli maneuver] for C-section/
Rupture clavicle or pubic symphysis

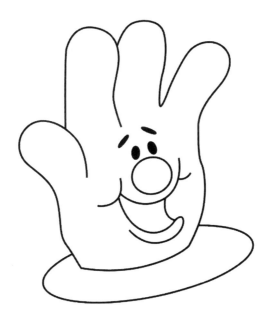

DYSTOCIA CAUSES
"4P's"

Passenger (large baby)
Passage (abnormal pelvis shape)
Propulsion (uterine contraction)
Proportion (disproportion Cephalo-pelvic)

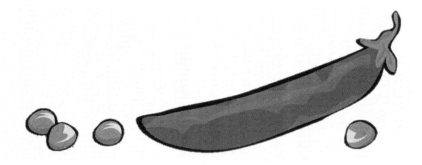

DYSTOCIA CAUSES
"3P's"

Power: strength of uterine contractions
Passage: size of the pelvic inlet and outlet
Passenger: the fetus--is it big, small, has anomalies, alive or dead?

Post-partum examination
"BUBBLES"

Breast
Uterus
Bowel
Bladder
Lochia
Episotomy
Surgical site (for Cesarean section)

Alternatively,
"BUBBLE HE"

Breast
Uterus
Bowel
Bladder
Lochia
Episiotomy

Homan's sign
Emotions

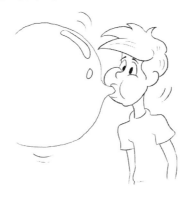

Developmental Stages (Embryology)
"Must Be Good"

Morula
Blastula
Gastrula

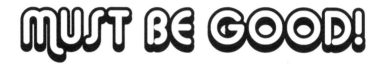

Definition of spontaneous abortion

"Spontaneous abortion" has **less than 20 letters** [it's exactly 19 letters].

"Spontaneous abortion" is defined as delivery or loss of products of conception at **less than 20 weeks** gestation.

Parity abbreviations (ie: G 2, P 0020)
"To Peace And Love"

T: of Term pregnancies
P: of Premature births
A: of Abortions (spontaneous or elective)
L: of Live births

- Describes the outcomes of the total number of pregnancies (Gravida).

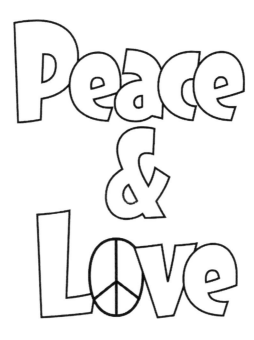

Indications of cesarean section
"MICE CAME"

M- Malpresentation
I- Induction failure
C- Cephalopelvic disproportion,contracted pelvis
E - Eclampsia
C- Cervical cancer
A- antepartum hemorrhage (Abruptio, placenta previa)
M- medical illness complicating pregnancy
E- Elderly primi (age > 35)

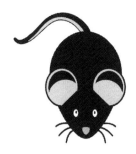

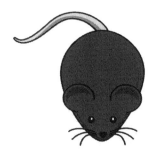

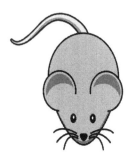

Cardiotocogram (CTG) interpretation
"Dr. C. BRaVADO"

Define **R**isk
Contractions (in 10 mins)
Baseline **R**ate (should be 110-160 bpm)
Variability (should be greater than 5)
Accelerations
Decelerations
Overall (normal or not)

PG E1 OR E2

CERVIPRIME HAS TWO Es SO IT MUST BE
PROSTAGLANDIN E2
MISOPROSTOL - PG E1

Cardinal movements of the fetus
"Don't Forget, I Enjoy Really Expensive Equipment"

Descent
Flexion
Internal rotation
Extension
Restitution
External rotation
Expulsion

Chapter 8
BABY/Toddler Milestones

APGAR score components
"SHIRT"

Skin color: blue or pink
Heart rate: below 100 or over 100
Irritability (response to stimulation): none, grimace or cry
Respirations: irregular or good
Tone (muscle): some flexion or active

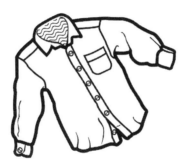

Alternatively,

APGAR score components
"APGAR"

Appearance: cyanosis--peripheral, central, none
Pulse: pulse rate
Grimace: response to stimulation
Activity: movement of the baby (muscle tone)
Respiration: respiratory rate

Alternatively,
APGAR score components
"5B's"

Breathing (respiratory effort)
Beating (heart rate)
Buff (tone)
Bothered (response to stimulation)
Blue (cyanosis)

Successive steps of neonatal resuscitation

"**D**o **W**hat **P**ediatricians **S**ay **T**o, **O**r **B**e **I**nviting **C**ostly **M**alpractice"

Drying
Warming
Positioning
Suctioning
Tactile stimulation
Oxygen
Bagging
Intubate endotracheally
Chest compressions
Medications

Perez reflex

Eliciting the **PErEz** reflex will make the baby **PEE**.

Fetal Head Diameter
(from smallest to largest)
M T P

Bi-**M**astoid-7.5
Bi-**T**emporal-8.00
Bi-**P**arietal-8.5

Head circumference by age

Remember **3**, **9**, and multiples of **5**:
Newborn **35** cm
3 mos **40** cm
9 mos **45** cm
3 yrs **50** cm
9 yrs **55**cm

When does birth weight double, triple, & quadruple?
Remember the124 1224 rule

1 day   birth wt
2 week   regain birth wt
4 month   **2x** birth wt
12 month   **3x** birth wt
24 month   **4x** birth wt

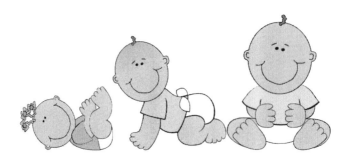

Average weights of children with age

Newborn **6** lbs
6 mos **12 lbs** (2x birth wt at 6 mos)
1 yr **18** (3x birth wt at 1 yr)
3 yrs **33** lbs
5 yrs **44 lbs**
7 yrs **55 lbs**
9 yrs **66 lbs**
11 yrs **77 lbs** (add 10 kg thereafter)
13 yrs **99 lbs**
15 yrs **121 lbs**
17 yrs **143 lbs**

Whey and Casein

Casein is more prominent in **C**ows milk and **W**hey is more prominent in **W**omen.
Breast milk is 30% casein / 70% whey
Cows milk is 80% casein / 20% whey
Whey is more easily digested and casein is more constipating.

Breast milk and breastfeeding jaundice

"Breastfeeding First"
Breastfeeding jaundice is the #1 cause of unconjugated hyperbilirubinemia and occurs in the **first week after birth.**
In breastfeeding jaundice the problem is not the milk, but how much feeding is occuring. The elevated bilirubin is due to low volume feeding exaggerating the physiologic jaundice by slow

gut movement increasing the enterohepatic circulation which in turn, causes dehydration.

Breast milk jaundice appears later, in days **6-14,** etiology is not certain but may include enzymatic inhibition of bilirubin conjugation.

Contraindicated drugs in breastfeeding "BREAST"

Bromocriptine/ **B**enzodiazepines
Radioactive isotopes/ **R**izatriptan
Ergotamine/ **E**thosuximide
Amiodarone/ **A**mphetamines
Stimulant laxatives/ **S**ex hormones
Tetracycline/ **T**retinoin

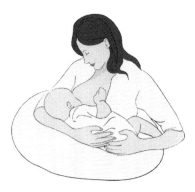

Risk factors for developmental dysplasia of the hip (DDH); Ortolani and Barlow

4 F's
First (firstborn)

Female (80% of all DDH)
Family history
Feet first (Breech).

For the first **four** months you need to ultrasound in order to confirm exam findings since the bones are not sufficiently ossified at this point to use x-ray.

Remember **Ortolani** goes **out** and **Barlow** pushes **back**. Short stature differential

"ABCDEFG"

Alone (neglected infant)
Bone dysplasias (rickets, scoliosis, mucopolysaccharidoses)
Chromosomal (Turner's, Down's)
Delayed growth
Endocrine (low growth hormone, Cushing's, hypothyroid)
Familial
GI malabsorption (celiac, Crohn's)

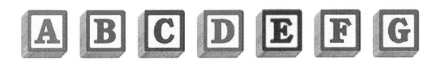

Midparental height

Remember 13 cm and that boys are taller than girls.
Boy = Average of parents + 13 cm
Girl = Average of parents - 13 cm

Pediatric development milestones

1 year: **single** words
2 years: **2** word sentences -understands **2** step commands
3 years: **3** word combos -repeats **3** digits -rides a **tri**cycle
4 years: draws **square (4 sides)**, counts **4** objects

Early development milestones

of blocks stacked = age in years
2 word sentences at 2
"Pee at three"; tricycle at three
"Four-square at four"= can hop at four
Drawings:
3yo= circle
4yo= cross
5yo= square
6yo=triangle

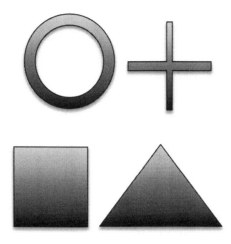

...more milestones

1 year:
Single words

2 years:
Climb 2 steps
2 word sentences
"Parallel" requires 2 things

3 years:
Tricycle.
Repeats 3 digits

4 years:
Copies a cross [4 points]
Shape copying:

Shapes are in alphabetical order: Circle(3yr),
Cross(4yr), Square(5yr), Triangle(6yr).

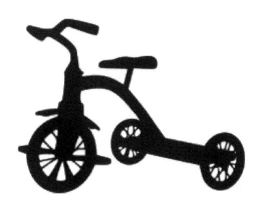

Dentition: eruption times of permanent dentition

"Mama **Is In P**ain, **P**apa **C**an **M**ake **M**edicine"
1st **M**olar: **6** years
1st **I**ncisor: **7** years
2nd **I**ncisor: **8** years
1st **P**remolar: **9** years
2nd **P**remolar: **10** years
Canine: **11** years
2nd **M**olar: **12** years
3rd **M**olar: 18-25 years

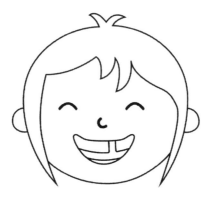

REFERENCES

http://www.fpnotebook.com/Gyn/Lab/PpSmr.htm

http://www.mcatprep.net/mnemMCAT.html

http://www.hopkinsmedicine.org/healthlibrary/conditions/gynecological_health/glossary_-_gynecological_health_85,P00562/

worldofmedicalmnemonics.blogspot.com/2008/08/obstetric-mnemonic.html

http://www.medicalgeek.com/mnemonics/10748-obstetrics-mnemonics-biggest-collection.html

http://familymed.uthscsa.edu/residency/maternityguide/abbreviations.htm

http://pediatricmnemonics.blogspot.com/2013/05/whey-and-casein.ht

http://pediatricmnemonics.blogspot.com/2013/12/when-does-birth-weight-double-triple.html

http://pediatricmnemonics.blogspot.com/2013/05/breast-milk-and-bre

http://pediatricmnemonics.blogspot.com/2012/12/ddh-risk-factors-m

http://pediatricmnemonics.blogspot.com/2013/12/midparental-heig

Other Books by Nachole Johnson

Medical Mnemonics for the Family Nurse Practitioner

NP School and Beyond: Tips for the Student Nurse Practitioner

The Financially Savvy Nurse Practitioner: Your Guide to Building Wealth

50+ Business Ideas For The Entrepreneurial Nurse

You're a Nurse and Want to Start Your Own Business? The Complete Guide

Adult-Gero and Family Nurse Practitioner Certification Review: Labs For Primary Care

Adult-Gero and Family Nurse Practitioner Certification Review: Mental Health

Adult-Gero and Family Nurse Practitioner Certification Review: Cardiac

Adult-Gero and Family Nurse Practitioner Certification Review: Health Promotion

Adult-Gero and Family Nurse Practitioner Certification Review: Pulmonary

Adult-Gero and Family Nurse Practitioner Certification Review: Genitourinary and STDs

Adult-Gero and Family Nurse Practitioner Certification Review: Neuro

Adult-Gero Primary Care and Family *Nurse Practitioner Certification Review:* HEENT

Adult-Gero Primary Care and Family Nurse Practitioner Certification Review: Women's Health

Adult-Gero Primary Care and Family Nurse Practitioner
Certification Review: GI & Liver

 Student Nurse Clinical Notebook

Student Nurse Practitioner Clinical Notebook

Nachole's Amazon Author Page:

amazon.com/author/nacholejohnson

Nachole's Blog: www.renursingedu.com

Made in the USA
Las Vegas, NV
11 January 2024

84223935R10042